MEDITERR
DIET
COOKBOOK
FOR
BEGINNERS

JOHN HARISTON

DISCLAIMER

The information contained in the Book is for informational purposes only, and in no way constitutes the making of a diagnosis or prescription for treatment.
The information contained in this book is not intended and should not in any way replace the direct relationship doctor-patient or specialist examination.
It is recommended that you always seek the advice of your physician and/or specialists for any reported indication.

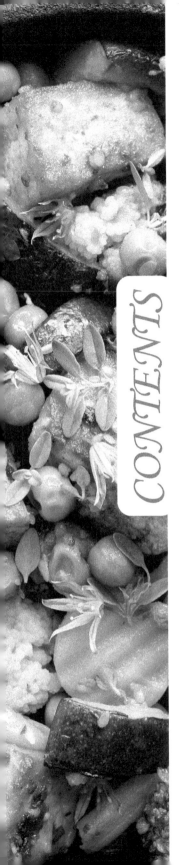

CONTENTS

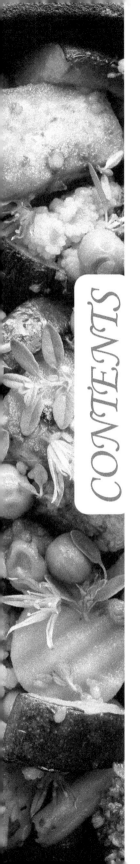

CONTENTS

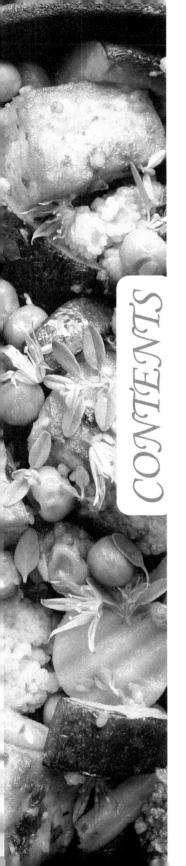

CONTENTS

Rice & Currant Salad Mediterranean Style

Servings: 4,

Cooking Time: 50 minutes

SHOPPING LIST:

- cup basmati rice salt

- 1/2 Tablespoons lemon juice 1 teaspoon grated orange zest

- 2 Tablespoons fresh orange juice 1/4 cup olive oil

- 1/2 teaspoon cinnamon

- Salt and pepper to taste 4 chopped green onions 1/2 cup dried currant

- 3/4 cup shelled pistachios or almonds 1/4 cup chopped fresh parsley

INSTRUCTIONS:

1. Place a non-stick pan over medium-high heat and add the rice. Toas the rice until it turns opaque and starts to smell, about 10 minutes.

2. Add 4 liters of boiling water to the pot and 2 teaspoons of salt. Bo until tender, about 8 minutes uncovered.

3. Drain the rice and spread it on a lined pan to cool completely.

4. In a large salad bowl, whisk the oil, juices and spices well. Add salt an pepper to taste.

5. Add half of the green onions, half of the parsley, currants and walnut

6. Season with the cooled rice and let it rest for at least 20 minutes.

. If necessary, season with pepper and salt.

. Garnish with the remaining parsley and green onions.

NUTRITIONAL VALUE:

Calories : 450

Carbs: 50.0g

Protein: 9.0g

Fat: 24.0g

Ricotta and Spinach Ravioli

Servings: 2,

Cooking Time: 15 minutes

SHOPPING LIST:

- 1 cup chicken stock

- 1 cup frozen spinach, thawed 1 batch pasta dough

- SHOPPING LIST: Filling

- 3 tbsp heavy cream 1 cup ricotta

- 1 ¾ cups baby spinach

- 1 small onion, finely chopped 2 tbsp butter

INSTRUCTIONS:

1. Prepare the filling: fry the onion and butter in a pan for about five minutes. Add the baby spinach leaves and continue to simmer for another four minutes. Remove from the heat, drain the liquid and chop the onion and leaves. Then combine with 2 tablespoons of cream and ricotta making sure it is well blended. Add pepper and salt to taste.

2. With the dough, divide it into four balls. Roll out a ball until you get a ¼-inch thick rectangular spread. Cut a 1½-inch by 3-inch rectangle. Place the filling in the center of the rectangles, about 1 tablespoon and brush the filling with cold water. Fold the rectangles in half, making sure there is no air trapped inside, and seal with a cookie cutter. Use all the filling.

3. Create the sauce for the pasta: until smooth, puree of chicken and

pinach broth. Pour into the heated pan and cook for two minutes. Add 1 ablespoon of cream and season with pepper and salt. Continue cooking or a minute and turn on the heat.

. Cook the ravioli by immersing them in a boiling pot of water with salt. ook until al dente then drain. Then quickly transfer the cooked ravioli to ae pasta sauce pan, mix to mix and serve.

NUTRITIONAL VALUE:

alories : 443

arbs: 12.3g

rotein: 18.8g

at: 36.8g

Roasted Red Peppers and Shrimp Pasta

Servings: 6,

Cooking Time: 10 minutes

SHOPPING LIST:

- 12 oz pasta, cooked and drained

- 1 cup finely shredded Parmesan Cheese

- ¼ cup snipped fresh basil

- ½ cup whipping cream

- ½ cup dry white wine

- 1 12oz jar roasted red sweet peppers, drained and chopped

- ¼ tsp crushed red pepper 6 cloves garlic, minced

- 1/3 cup finely chopped onion 2 tbsp olive oil

- ¼ cup butter

- 1 ½ lbs. fresh, peeled, deveined, rinsed and drained medium shrimps

INSTRUCTIONS:

1. Over medium-high heat, heat the butter in a large skillet and add th garlic and onions. Stir until the onions are soft, about two minutes. Ad chopped red pepper and shrimp, sauté for another two minutes befor adding wine and roasted peppers.

2. Allow the mixture to boil before lowering the heat to low heat an

immer without a lid for two minutes. Stirring occasionally, add the cream nce the shrimp are cooked and simmer for a minute.

. Add the basil and remove from the heat. Add the pasta and mix gently. ransfer to serving plates and garnish with cheese.

NUTRITIONAL VALUE:

alories : 418

arbs: 26.9g

rotein: 37.1g

at: 18.8g

Seafood and Veggie Pasta

Servings: 4,

Cooking Time: 20 minutes

SHOPPING LIST:

- ¼ tsp pepper
- ¼ tsp salt
- 1 lb raw shelled shrimp 1 lemon, cut into wedges 1 tbsp butter
- tbsp olive oil
- 5-oz cans chopped clams, drained (reserve 2 tbsp clam juice) 2 tbs dry white wine
- 4 cloves garlic, minced
- 4 cups zucchini, spiraled (use a veggie spiralizer) 4 tbsp Parmesa Cheese
- Chopped fresh parsley to garnish

INSTRUCTIONS:

1. Prepare the courgettes and spiral with a vegetarian spiralizer. Arrang 1 cup of zucchini noodles per bowl. Total of 4 bowls.

2. Over medium heat, place a large non-stick saucepan and heat oil an butter.

3. For one minute, sauté the garlic. Add the shrimp and cook for 3 minute until opaque or cooked through.

4. Add the white wine, the clam juice kept aside and the clams. Bring t

boil and continue to simmer for 2 minutes or until half of the liquid has vaporated. Stir continuously.

. Season with pepper and salt. And if necessary add more to taste.

. Remove from heat and distribute the seafood sauce evenly in 4 bowls.

. Top with a tablespoon of Parmesan per bowl, serve and enjoy.

NUTRITIONAL VALUE:

Calories : 324.9; Carbs: 12g; Protein: 43.8g; Fat: 11.3g

Simple Penne Anti-Pasto

Servings: 4,

Cooking Time: 15 minutes

SHOPPING LIST:

- ½ cup whole wheat couscous

- 4 oz small shrimp, peeled and deveined 4 oz bay scallops, tough muscle removed

- ¼ cup vegetable broth

- 1 cup freshly diced tomatoes and juice Pinch of crumbled saffron threads

- ¼ tsp freshly ground pepper

- ¼ tsp salt

- ½ tsp fennel seed

- ½ tsp dried thyme

- 1 clove garlic, minced

- 1 medium onion, chopped 2 tsp extra virgin olive oil

INSTRUCTIONS:

1. Place a large saucepan over medium heat and add the oil. Stir in the onion and sauté for three minutes before adding: saffron, pepper, salt, fennel seeds, thyme and garlic. Continue to brown for another minute.

2. Then add the broth and tomatoes and bring to a boil. Once boiled reduce the heat, cover and continue cooking for another 2 minutes.

. Add the scallops and increase the heat to medium, stir occasionally nd cook for two minutes. Add the shrimp and wait another two minutes efore adding the couscous. Then remove from heat, cover and set aside or five minutes before mixing thoroughly.

NUTRITIONAL VALUE:

Calories : 117; Carbs: 11.7g; Protein: 11.5g; Fat: 3.1g

Shrimp Paella Made with Quinoa

Servings: 7,

Cooking Time: 40 minutes

SHOPPING LIST:

- 1 lb. large shrimp, peeled, deveined and thawed 1 tsp seafood seasonin
- 1 cup frozen green peas
- 1 red bell pepper, cored, seeded & membrane removed, sliced into ½ strips
- ½ cup sliced sun-dried tomatoes, packed in olive oil Salt to taste
- ½ tsp black pepper
- ½ tsp Spanish paprika
- ½ tsp saffron threads (optional turmeric) 1 bay leaf
- ¼ tsp crushed red pepper flakes
- 3 cups chicken broth, fat free, low sodium 1 ½ cups dry quinoa, rins well
- tbsp olive oil
- cloves garlic, minced 1 yellow onion, diced

INSTRUCTIONS:

1. Season the prawns with sea sauce and a pinch of salt. Stir to mix wel and refrigerate until use.

2. Prepare and wash the quinoa. To put aside.

. Over medium-low heat, place a large non-stick pan and heat the oil. dd the onions and sauté for 5 minutes until soft and tender.

. Add the paprika, saffron (or turmeric), bay leaves, chilli flakes, chicken roth and quinoa. Season with salt and pepper.

. Cover the pan and bring to a boil. Once it boils, lower the heat to a boil nd cook until all the liquid is absorbed, about ten minutes.

. Add the prawns, peas and dried tomatoes. Cover and cook for 5 minutes.

. Once done, turn off the heat and let the paella solidify for ten minutes hile still covered.

. To serve, remove the bay leaf and enjoy with a squeeze of lemon if esired.

NUTRITIONAL VALUE:

alories : 324.4; Protein: 22g; Carbs: 33g; Fat: 11.6g

Shrimp, Lemon and Basil Pasta

Servings: 4,

Cooking Time: 25 minutes

SHOPPING LIST:

- 2 cups baby spinach
- ½ tsp salt
- 2 tbsp fresh lemon juice
- 2 tbsp extra virgin olive oil 3 tbsp drained capers
- ¼ cup chopped fresh basil
- 1 lb. peeled and deveined large shrimp 8 oz uncooked spaghetti
- 3 quarts water

INSTRUCTIONS:

1. In a saucepan, bring 3 liters of water to a boil. Add the pasta and bo for another eight minutes before adding the shrimp and boil for anothe three minutes or until the pasta is cooked.

2. Drain the pasta and transfer it to a bowl. Add the salt, lemon juice, oliv oil, capers and basil, mixing well.

3. To serve, place the baby spinach on a plate for about ½ cup and to with ½ cup of pasta.

NUTRITIONAL VALUE:

Calories : 151; Carbs: 18.9g; Protein: 4.3g; Fat: 7.4g

Simple Penne Anti-Pasto

Servings: 4,

Cooking Time: 15 minutes

SHOPPING LIST:

¼ cup pine nuts, toasted

½ cup grated Parmigiano-Reggiano cheese, divided 8oz penne pasta, cooked and drained

1 6oz jar drained, sliced, marinated and quartered artichoke hearts

1 7 oz jar drained and chopped sun-dried tomato halves packed in oil 3 oz chopped prosciutto

1/3 cup pesto

½ cup pitted and chopped Kalamata olives 1 medium red bell pepper

INSTRUCTIONS:

. Slice the pepper, discard the membranes, seeds and stem. On an aluminum-lined pan, place the pepper halves, press by hand and bake in the oven for eight minutes. Remove from the oven, place in a sealed bag for 5 minutes before peeling and mincing.

. Put the chopped pepper in a bowl and add the artichokes, tomatoes, ham, pesto and olives.

3. Add ¼ cup of cheese and pasta. Transfer to a serving dish and garnish with ¼ cup of cheese and pine nuts. Serve and enjoy!

NUTRITIONAL VALUE:

Calories : 606

Carbs: 70.3g

Protein: 27.2g

Fat: 27.6g

Spaghetti in Lemon Avocado White Sauce

ervings: 6,

ooking Time: 30 minutes

HOPPING LIST:

Freshly ground black pepper Zest and juice of 1 lemon

1 avocado, pitted and peeled 1-pound spaghetti

Salt

1 tbsp Olive oil

8 oz small shrimp, shelled and deveined

¼ cup dry white wine

large onion, finely sliced

NSTRUCTIONS:

. Boil a large pot of water. Once boiling add the spaghetti or pasta and ook following the manufacturer's instructions until al dente. Drain and et aside.

. In a large skillet, sauté the wine and onions over medium heat for ten ninutes or until the onions are translucent and soft.

. Add the shrimp to the pan and increase the heat to high while constantly rowning until the shrimp are cooked through about five minutes. Turn ff the heat. Season with salt and add the oil immediately. Then quickly kip the cooked pasta, mix well.

4. In a blender, until smooth, blend the lemon juice and avocado. Pour the pasta into the pan, combine well. Garnish with pepper and lemon zest and serve.

NUTRITIONAL VALUE:

Calories : 206

Carbs: 26.3g

Protein: 10.2g

Fat: 8.0g

Spanish Rice Casserole with Cheesy Beef

Servings: 2,

Cooking Time: 32 minutes

SHOPPING LIST:

tablespoons chopped green bell pepper 1/4 teaspoon Worcestershire sauce

1/4 teaspoon ground cumin

1/4 cup shredded Cheddar cheese 1/4 cup finely chopped onion

1/4 cup chile sauce

1/3 cup uncooked long grain rice 1/2-pound lean ground beef

1/2 teaspoon salt

1/2 teaspoon brown sugar

1/2 pinch ground black pepper 1/2 cup water

1/2 (14.5 ounce) can canned tomatoes 1 tablespoon chopped fresh cilantro

INSTRUCTIONS:

. Place a non-stick saucepan over medium heat and brown the meat for 0 minutes while crumbling the meat. Discard the fat.

. Mix the pepper, Worcestershire sauce, cumin, brown sugar, salt, chili sauce, rice, water, tomatoes, green pepper and onion. Mix well and cook or 10 minutes until blended and a little tender.

. Transfer to an ovenproof dish and press firmly. Sprinkle with cheese and bake for 7 minutes in a preheated 400oF oven. Cook for 3 minute until the top is lightly browned.

4. Serve and enjoy with chopped cilantro.

NUTRITIONAL VALUE:

Calories : 460

Carbohydrates: 35.8g

Protein: 37.8g

Fat: 17.9g

Squash and Eggplant Casserole

Servings: 2,

Cooking Time: 45 minutes

SHOPPING LIST:

½ cup dry white wine

1 eggplant, halved and cut to 1-inch slices 1 large onion, cut into wedges

1 red bell pepper, seeded and cut to julienned strips 1 small butternut squash, cut into 1-inch slices

 tbsp olive oil 12 baby corn

cups low sodium vegetable broth Salt and pepper to taste

Polenta Shopping List:

¼ cup parmesan cheese, grated 1 cup instant polenta

2 tbsp fresh oregano, chopped Topping Shopping List:

1 garlic clove, chopped 2 tbsp slivered almonds 5 tbsp parsley, chopped

Grated zest of 1 lemon

INSTRUCTIONS:

1. Preheat the oven to 350 degrees Fahrenheit.

2. In a saucepan, heat the oil and add the onion wedges and corn on th cob. Brown over medium-high heat for five minutes. Stir occasionally t prevent the onions and corn on the cob from sticking to the bottom of th pan.

3. Add the squash to the saucepan and mix the vegetables. Add th aubergines and chilli.

4. Cover the vegetables and cook over medium-low heat.

5. Cook for about ten minutes before adding the wine. Let the wine sizzl before adding the broth. Bring to a boil and cook in the oven for 3 minutes.

6. While the casserole is cooking inside the oven, cover by spreading th flaked almonds on a baking sheet and toasting under the wire rack unti lightly browned.

7. Put the toasted almonds in a small bowl and mix the rest of the shoppin list: for the fillings.

8. Prepare the polenta. In a large saucepan, bring 3 cups of water to a boi over high heat.

9. Add the polenta and continue beating until it has absorbed all the wate

10. Reduce the heat to medium temperature until the polenta is thick. Ad the parmesan and oregano.

1. Serve the polenta on plates and add over the saucepan. Sprinkle the toppings on top.

NUTRITIONAL VALUE:

Calories: 579.3

Carbs: 79.2g

Protein: 22.2g

Fat: 19.3g

Stuffed Tomatoes with Green Chili

Servings: 6,

Cooking Time: 55 minutes

SHOPPING LIST:

- 4 oz Colby-Jack shredded cheese
- ¼ cup water
- 1 cup uncooked quinoa 6 large ripe tomatoes
- ¼ tsp freshly ground black pepper
- ¾ tsp ground cumin 1 tsp salt, divided
- 1 tbsp fresh lime juice 1 tbsp olive oil
- tbsp chopped fresh oregano 1 cup chopped onion
- cups fresh corn kernels
- 2 poblano chilies

INSTRUCTIONS:

1. Preheat the grill to maximum.

2. Slice the peppers lengthwise and press them onto a tin lined pan. Gril for 8 minutes. Remove from the oven and let cool for 10 minutes. Peel th chillies and chop them coarsely and place them in a medium-sized bow.

3. Place the onion and corn in the pan and grill for ten minutes. Stir twic while grilling. Remove from the oven and mix with the chopped chillies

4. Add black pepper, cumin, ¼ teaspoon of salt, lime juice, oil an oregano. Mix well.

. Cut the tops of the tomatoes and set them aside. Leave the tomato shell ntact as you harvest the tomato pulp.

. Drain the tomato pulp by pressing with a spoon. Reserve 1 ¼ cup of quid tomato pulp and discard the rest. Turn the tomato shells upside own on a wire rack for 30 minutes and then pat the inside dry with a aper towel.

. Season the tomato pulp with ½ teaspoon of salt.

. On a colander over a bowl, place the quinoa. Add the water to cover the uinoa. Rub the quinoa grains for 30 seconds with your hands; rinse and rain. Repeat this procedure twice and drain well at the end.

. Bring the remaining salt, ¼ cup water, quinoa and tomato liquid to a oil in a medium saucepan.

0. Once it boils, reduce the heat and simmer for 15 minutes or until the quid is completely absorbed. Remove from the heat and peel the quinoa ith a fork. Transfer and mix the quinoa well with the corn mixture.

1. Pour ¾ cup of the quinoa and corn mixture into the tomato shells, over with the cheese and cover with the top of the tomato. Bake in a reheated 350 ° F oven for 15 minutes and then broil for another 1.5 ninutes.

NUTRITIONAL VALUE:

Calories: 276; Carbs: 46.3g; Protein: 13.4g; Fat: 4.1g

Tasty Lasagna Rolls

Servings: 6,

Cooking Time: 20 minutes

SHOPPING LIST:

- ¼ tsp crushed red pepper
- ¼ tsp salt
- ½ cup shredded mozzarella cheese
- ½ cups parmesan cheese, shredded 1 14-oz package tofu, cubed
- 1 25-oz can of low-sodium marinara sauce 1 tbsp extra virgin olive o
- 12 whole wheat lasagna noodles 2 tbsp Kalamata olives, chopped cloves minced garlic
- 3 cups spinach, chopped

INSTRUCTIONS:

1. Put enough water in a large pot and cook the lasagna according to th instructions on the package. Drain, rinse and set aside until use.

2. In a large skillet, sauté the garlic over medium heat for 20 second Add the tofu and spinach and cook until the spinach wilt. Transfer thi mixture to a bowl and add the Parmesan, olives, salt, chilli and 2/3 cup c marinara sauce.

3. Spread a cup of marinara sauce on the bottom in a pan. To make th rolls, place the noodles on a surface and sprinkle ¼ cup of the tofu filling Roll it up and place it on the pan with the marinara sauce. Do this until a the lasagna is rolled up.

. Put the pan over high heat and bring to a boil. Reduce the heat to medium and let it cook for another three minutes. Sprinkle the mozzarella nd let the cheese melt for two minutes. Serve hot.

NUTRITIONAL VALUE:

Calories : 304

Carbs: 39.2g

Protein: 23g

Fat: 19.2g

Tasty Mushroom Bolognese

Servings: 6,

Cooking Time: 65 minutes

SHOPPING LIST:

- ¼ cup chopped fresh parsley
- oz Parmigiano-Reggiano cheese, grated 1 tbsp kosher salt
- 10-oz whole wheat spaghetti, cooked and drained
- ¼ cup milk
- 14-oz can whole peeled tomatoes
- ½ cup white wine
- tbsp tomato paste
- 1 tbsp minced garlic
- 8 cups finely chopped cremini mushrooms
- ½ lb. ground pork
- ½ tsp freshly ground black pepper, divided
- ¾ tsp kosher salt, divided 2 ½ cups chopped onion 1 tbsp olive oil
- 1 cup boiling water
- ½-oz dried porcini mushrooms

INSTRUCTIONS:

1. Let the mushrooms rest in a bowl of boiling water for twenty minutes drain (reserve the liquid), rinse and chop. To put aside.

. Over medium-high heat, place a Dutch oven with olive oil and cook for
:n minutes cook the pork, ¼ teaspoon of pepper, ¼ teaspoon of salt and
nions. Stir constantly to break up the ground pork pieces.

. Mix ¼ teaspoon of pepper, ¼ teaspoon of salt, garlic and cremini
ushrooms. Continue cooking until the liquid has evaporated, about
fteen minutes.

. Stirring constantly, add the mushrooms and sauté for a minute.

. Mix the wine, the boletus liquid, the tomatoes and the tomato paste. Let
 simmer for forty minutes. Stir occasionally. Pour in the milk and cook
or another two minutes before removing from the heat.

. Incorporate the pasta and transfer it to a serving dish. Garnish with
arsley and cheese before serving.

NUTRITIONAL VALUE:

alories : 358; Carbs: 32.8g; Protein: 21.1g; Fat: 15.4g

Tortellini Salad with Broccoli

Servings: 12,

Cooking Time: 20 minutes

SHOPPING LIST:

- 1 red onion, chopped finely 1 cup sunflower seeds

- 1 cup raisins

- 3 heads fresh broccoli, cut into florets 2 tsp cider vinegar

- ½ cup white sugar

- ½ cup mayonnaise

- 20-oz fresh cheese filled tortellini

INSTRUCTIONS:

1. In a large pot of boiling water, cook the tortellini according to th manufacturer's instructions. Drain and rinse with cold water and set aside

2. Whisk the vinegar, sugar, and mayonnaise to create the salad dressing

3. Mix the red onion, sunflower seeds, raisins, tortellini and broccoli in large bowl. Pour in the dressing and mix to coat.

4. Serve and enjoy.

NUTRITIONAL VALUE:

Calories : 272; Carbs: 38.7g; Protein: 5.0g; Fat: 8.1g

Turkey and Quinoa Stuffed Peppers

Servings: 6,

Cooking Time: 55 minutes

SHOPPING LIST:

3 large red bell peppers

tsp chopped fresh rosemary 2 tbsp chopped fresh parsley

tbsp chopped pecans, toasted

¼ cup extra virgin olive oil

½ cup chicken stock

½ lb. fully cooked smoked turkey sausage, diced

½ tsp salt

2 cups water

cup uncooked quinoa

INSTRUCTIONS:

. Over high heat, put a large pot and add salt, water and quinoa. Bring to the boil.

. Once it boils, reduce the heat to a boil, cover and cook until all the water is absorbed about 15 minutes.

. Uncover the quinoa, turn off the heat and let it rest for another 5 minutes.

. Add the rosemary, parsley, pecans, olive oil, chicken broth, and turkey sausage to the quinoa pan. Mix well.

5. Cut the peppers in half lengthwise and discard the membranes an seeds. In another pot of boiling water, add the peppers, boil for 5 minutes drain and discard the water.

6. Grease a 13 x 9 pan and preheat the oven to 350oF.

7. Place the boiled pepper on the prepared baking sheet, fill evenly wit the quinoa mixture and place in the oven.

Bake for 15 minutes.

NUTRITIONAL VALUE:

Calories : 255.6; Carbs: 21.6g; Protein: 14.4g; Fat: 12.4g

Veggie Pasta with Shrimp, Basil and Lemon

Servings: 4,

Cooking Time: 5 minutes

SHOPPING LIST:

cups baby spinach

½ tsp salt

2 tbsp fresh lemon juice

2 tbsp extra virgin olive oil 3 tbsp drained capers

¼ cup chopped fresh basil

lb. peeled and deveined large shrimp 4 cups zucchini, spirals

INSTRUCTIONS:

. divide into 4 serving plates, top with ¼ cup of spinach, serve and enjoy.

NUTRITIONAL VALUE:

Calories : 51

Carbs: 4.4g

Protein: 1.8g

Fat: 3.4g

Veggies and Sun-Dried Tomato Alfredo

Servings: 4,

Cooking Time: 30 minutes

SHOPPING LIST:

- tsp finely shredded lemon peel
- ½ cup finely shredded Parmesan cheese 1 ¼ cups milk
- 2 tbsp all-purpose flour
- 8 fresh mushrooms, sliced
- 1 ½ cups fresh broccoli florets
- 4 oz fresh trimmed and quartered Brussels sprouts 4 oz trimmed fresh asparagus spears
- 1 tbsp olive oil 4 tbsp butter
- ½ cup chopped dried tomatoes 8 oz dried fettuccine

INSTRUCTIONS:

1. In a pot of boiling water, add the fettuccine and cook according to the manufacturer's instructions. Two minutes before the pasta is cooked, add the dried tomatoes. Drain the pasta and tomatoes and put them back in the pot to keep them warm. To put aside.

2. Over medium-high heat, in a large skillet with 1 tablespoon of butter, sauté the mushrooms, broccoli, Brussels sprouts and asparagus. Cook covered for eight minutes, transfer to a plate and set aside.

3. Using the same pan, add the remaining butter and flour. Stirring

igorously, cook for one minute or until thickened. Add the Parmesan, milk and stir until the cheese has melted about five minutes.

. Add the pasta and mix. Transfer to serving dish. Garnish with Parmesan nd lemon zest before serving.

NUTRITIONAL VALUE:

Calories : 439

Carbs: 52.0g

Protein: 16.3g

Fat: 19.5g

Yangchow Chinese Style Fried Rice

Servings: 4,

Cooking Time: 20 minutes

SHOPPING LIST:

- 4 cups cold cooked rice 1/2 cup peas

- 1 medium yellow onion, diced 5 tbsp olive oil

- 4 oz frozen medium shrimp, thawed, shelled, deveined and choppe finely 6 oz roast pork

- large eggs

- Salt and freshly ground black pepper 1/2 tsp cornstarch

INSTRUCTIONS:

1. Combine the salt and ground black pepper and 1/2 teaspoon c cornstarch, sprinkle the shrimp with it. Chop the roast pork. Beat the egg and set them aside.

2. Stir the shrimp in a wok over high heat with 1 tablespoon of heated o until pink, about 3 minutes. Set the shrimp aside and briefly fry the roas pork. Remove both from the pan.

3. In the same pan, sauté the onion until soft, stir in the peas and coo until bright green. Remove both from the pan.

4. Add 2 tablespoons of oil to the same pan, add the cooked rice. Mix an

parate the individual beans. Add the beaten eggs, skip the rice. Add the
asted pork, shrimp, vegetables and onion. Put it all together. Season
ith salt and pepper to taste.

NUTRITIONAL VALUE:

alories : 556

arbs: 60.2g

rotein: 20.2g

at: 25.2g

Rustic Lentil-Rice Pilaf

Prep time: 5 minutes | Cook time: 50 minutes | Serves 6

Shopping List:

- ¼ cup extra-virgin olive oil

- 1 large onion, chopped

- 6 cups water

- 1 teaspoon ground cumin

- 1 teaspoon salt

- 2 cups brown lentils, picked over and rinsed

- 1 cup basmati rice

Instructions:

1. In a medium saucepan over medium heat, cook the olive oil and onion for 7-10 minutes until the edges are golden.

2. Raise the heat, add the water, cumin and salt and bring the mixture to boil, boiling for about 3 minutes.

3. Add the lentils and reduce the heat to medium-low. Cover the pot an cook for 20 minutes, stirring occasionally.

. Incorporate the rice and cover; cook for another 20 minutes.

. Fluff the rice with a fork and serve hot.

Nutritional Value:

Calories: 397

Fat: 11g

Protein: 18g

Carbs: 60g

Fiber: 18g

Sodium: 396mg

Bulgur Pilaf with Garbanzos

Prep time: 5 minutes | Cook time: 20 minutes | Serves 4 to 6

Shopping List:

- 3 tablespoons extra-virgin olive oil

- 1 large onion, chopped

- 1 (16-ounce / 454-g) can garbanzo beans, rinsed and drained

- 2 cups bulgur wheat, rinsed and drained

- 1½ teaspoons salt

- ½ teaspoon cinnamon

- 4 cups water

Instructions:

1. In a large saucepan over medium heat, cook the olive oil and onion for 5 minutes.

2. Add the chickpeas and cook for another 5 minutes.

3. Add the bulgur, salt, cinnamon and water and mix to combine. Cover the pot, lower the heat and cook for 10 minutes.

4. When cooking is finished, puff the pilaf with a fork. Cover and let it rest for another 5 minutes.

Nutritional Value:

calories: 462 | fat: 13g | protein: 15g | carbs: 76g | fiber: 19g | sodium 890mg

Lentil Bulgur Pilaf

Prep time: 10 minutes | Cook time: 50 minutes | Serves 6

Shopping List:

½ cup extra-virgin olive oil

4 large onions, chopped

2 teaspoons salt, divided

6 cups water

2 cups brown lentils, picked over and rinsed

1 teaspoon freshly ground black pepper

1 cup bulgur wheat

Instructions:

. In a large saucepan over medium heat, cook and mix the olive oil, onions and 1 teaspoon of salt for 12-15 minutes, until the onions turn a medium brown / golden color.

. Place half of the cooked onions in a bowl.

. Add the water, the remaining 1 teaspoon of salt and the lentils to the remaining onions. Shake. Cover and cook for 30 minutes.

4. Mix the black pepper and bulgur, cover and cook for 5 minutes. Fluf with a fork, cover and let sit for another 5 minutes.

5. Pour the lentils and bulgur onto a serving dish and garnish with the se aside onions. Serve hot.

Nutritional Value:

calories: 479 | fat: 20g | protein: 20g | carbs: 60g | fiber: 24g | sodium 789mg

Simple Spanish Rice

Prep time: 10 minutes | Cook time: 20 minutes | Serves 4

Shopping List:

2 tablespoons extra-virgin olive oil

1 medium onion, finely chopped

1 large tomato, finely diced

2 tablespoons tomato paste

1 teaspoon smoked paprika

1 teaspoon salt

1½ cups basmati rice

3 cups water

Instructions:

1. In a medium saucepan over medium heat, cook the olive oil, onion and tomato for 3 minutes.

2. Incorporate the tomato paste, paprika, salt and rice. Cook for 1 minute.

3. Add the water, cover the pot and reduce the heat. Cook for 12 minutes.

4. Gently flip the rice, cover and cook for another 3 minutes.

Nutritional Value:

Calories: 328 | fat: 7g | protein: 6g | carbs: 60g | fiber: 2g | sodium: 651mg

Creamy Parmesan Garlic Polenta

Prep time: 5 minutes | Cook time: 30 minutes | Serves 4

Shopping List:

- 4 tablespoons (½ stick) unsalted butter, divided (optional)
- 1 tablespoon garlic, finely chopped
- 4 cups water
- 1 teaspoon salt
- 1 cup polenta
- ¾ cup Parmesan cheese, divided

Instructions:

1. In a large saucepan over medium heat, cook 3 tablespoons of butter (: desired) and garlic for 2 minutes.

2. Add the water and salt and bring to a boil. Add the polenta and blen immediately until it begins to thicken, about 3 minutes. Lower the hea cover and cook for 25 minutes, whisking every 5 minutes.

3. Using a wooden spoon, stir in ½ cup of Parmesan.

4. To serve, pour the polenta into a large serving bowl. Sprinkle the to with the remaining 1 tablespoon of butter (if desired) and ¼ cup of th remaining Parmesan. Serve hot.

Nutritional Value:

calories: 297 | fat: 16g | protein: 9g | carbs: 28g | fiber: 2g | sodium: 838m

Mushroom Parmesan Risotto

Prep time: 10 minutes | Cook time: 30 minutes | Serves 4

Shopping List:

6 cups vegetable broth

3 tablespoons extra-virgin olive oil, divided

1 pound (454 g) cremini mushrooms, cleaned and sliced

1 medium onion, finely chopped

2 cloves garlic, minced

1½ cups Arborio rice

1 teaspoon salt

½ cup freshly grated Parmesan cheese

½ teaspoon freshly ground black pepper

Instructions:

. In a saucepan over medium heat, bring the broth over low heat.

. In a large skillet over medium heat, cook 1 tablespoon of olive oil and sliced mushrooms for 5-7 minutes. Set the cooked mushrooms aside.

. In the same pan over medium heat, add the remaining 2 tablespoons of olive oil, onion and garlic. Cook for 3 minutes.

. Add the rice, salt and 1 cup of broth to the pan. Mix the shopping list:

together and cook over low heat until most of the liquid is absorbed. Continue adding ½ cup of broth at a time, stirring until completely absorbed. Repeat until all the broth is used up.

5. With the last addition of broth, add the cooked mushrooms, Parmesan and black pepper. Cook for another 2 minutes. Serve immediately.

Nutritional Value:

calories: 410 | fat: 12g | protein: 11g | carbs: 65g | fiber: 3g | sodium 2086mg

Brown Rice Bowls with Roasted Vegetables

Prep time: 15 minutes | Cook time: 20 minutes | Serves 4

Shopping List:

Nonstick cooking spray

2 cups broccoli florets

2 cups cauliflower florets

1 (15-ounce / 425-g) can chickpeas, drained and rinsed

1 cup carrots sliced 1 inch thick

2 to 3 tablespoons extra-virgin olive oil, divided

Salt and freshly ground black pepper, to taste

2 to 3 tablespoons sesame seeds, for garnish

2 cups cooked brown rice

Dressing:

3 to 4 tablespoons tahini

2 tablespoons honey

1 lemon, juiced

1 garlic clove, minced

Salt and freshly ground black pepper, to taste

Instructions:

1. Preheat the oven to 400°F (205°C). Spray two baking sheets wit cooking spray.

2. Cover the first pan with the broccoli and cauliflower and the secon with the chickpeas and carrots. Season each sheet with half the oil an season with salt and pepper before baking.

3. Cook the carrots and chickpeas for 10 minutes, leaving the carrots sti just crispy, the broccoli and cauliflower for 20 minutes, until tender. Sti each halfway through cooking.

4. To prepare the dressing, in a small bowl, blend the tahini, honey, lemo juice and garlic. Season with salt and pepper and set aside.

5. Divide the rice into individual bowls, then sprinkle with vegetables an season with seasoning on the plate.

Nutritional Value:

calories: 454 | fat: 18g | protein: 12g | carbs: 62g | fiber: 11g | sodium 61mg

Spanish Chicken and Rice

Prep time: 15 minutes | Cook time: 30 minutes | Serves 2

Shopping List:

2 teaspoons smoked paprika

2 teaspoons ground cumin

1½ teaspoons garlic salt

¾ teaspoon chili powder

¼ teaspoon dried oregano

1 lemon

2 boneless, skinless chicken breasts

3 tablespoons extra-virgin olive oil, divided

2 large shallots, diced

1 cup uncooked white rice

2 cups vegetable stock

1 cup broccoli florets

⅓ cup chopped parsley

Instructions:

1. In a small bowl, whisk together the paprika, cumin, garlic salt, chili powder, and oregano. Divide in half and set aside. In another small bowl, squeeze the lemon and set aside.

2. Place the chicken in a medium bowl. Sprinkle the chicken with 2

tablespoons of olive oil and scrub with half of the seasoning mixture.

3. In a large skillet, heat the remaining 1 tablespoon of olive oil and coo the chicken for 2 to 3 minutes on each side, until just golden but cooke through.

4. Add the shallot to the same pan and cook until translucent, then add th rice and cook for another minute to toast. Add the vegetable stock, lemo juice, and remaining seasoning mixture and toss to combine. Return th chicken to the pan on top of the rice. Cover and cook for 15 minutes.

5. Uncover and add the broccoli florets. Cover and cook for another minutes, until the liquid is absorbed, the rice is tender, and the chicken i cooked through.

6. Top with freshly chopped parsley and serve immediately.

Nutritional Value:

calories: 750 | fat: 25g | protein: 36g | carbs: 101g | fiber: 7g | sodium 1823mg

Mushroom Barley Pilaf

Prep time: 5 minutes | Cook time: 37 minutes | Serves 4

Shopping List:

Olive oil cooking spray

2 tablespoons olive oil

8 ounces (227 g) button mushrooms, diced

½ yellow onion, diced

2 garlic cloves, minced

1 cup pearl barley

2 cups vegetable broth

1 tablespoon fresh thyme, chopped

½ teaspoon salt

¼ teaspoon smoked paprika

Fresh parsley, for garnish

Instructions:

. Preheat the air fryer to 380°F (193°C). Lightly coat the inside of a -cup saucepan with cooking spray olive oil. (The shape of the saucepan will depend on the size of the air fryer, but it must be able to hold at least cups.)

. In a large skillet, heat the olive oil over medium heat. Add the mushrooms and onion and cook, stirring occasionally, for 5 minutes or until the mushrooms begin to brown.

3. Add the garlic and cook for another 2 minutes. Transfer the vegetable to a large bowl.

4. Add the barley, stock, thyme, salt and paprika.

5. Pour the barley and vegetable mixture into the prepared saucepan and place the dish in the air fryer. Bake for 15 minutes.

6. Stir in the barley mixture. Reduce the heat to 182 ° C, then return the barley to the air fryer and bake for another 15 minutes.

7. Remove from air fryer and let sit for 5 minutes before blending with fork and garnish with fresh parsley.

Nutritional Value:

calories: 263 | fat: 8g | protein: 7g | carbs: 44g | fiber: 9g | sodium: 576mg

Toasted Barley and Almond Pilaf

Prep time: 10 minutes | Cook time: 5 minutes | Serves 2

Shopping List:

1 tablespoon olive oil

1 garlic clove, minced

3 scallions, minced

2 ounces (57 g) mushrooms, sliced

¼ cup sliced almonds

½ cup uncooked pearled barley

1½ cups low-sodium chicken stock

½ teaspoon dried thyme

1 tablespoon fresh minced parsley

Salt, to taste

Instructions:

. Heat the oil in a saucepan over medium-high heat. Add the garlic, shallots, mushrooms and almonds and sauté for 3 minutes.

. Add the barley and cook, stirring, for 1 minute to toast.

. Add the chicken stock and thyme and bring the mixture to a boil.

4. Cover and reduce heat to low. Boil the barley for 30 minutes or until the liquid is absorbed and the barley is tender.

5. Sprinkle with fresh parsley and season with salt before serving.

Nutritional Value:

calories: 333 | fat: 13g | protein: 10g | carbs: 46g | fiber: 9g | sodium 141mg

Mediterranean Lentils and Brown Rice

Prep time: 15 minutes | Cook time: 23 minutes | Serves 4

Shopping List:

2¼ cups low-sodium or no-salt-added vegetable broth

½ cup uncooked brown or green lentils

½ cup uncooked instant brown rice

½ cup diced carrots

½ cup diced celery

1 (2¼-ounce / 64-g) can sliced olives, drained

¼ cup diced red onion

¼ cup chopped fresh curly-leaf parsley

1½ tablespoons extra-virgin olive oil

1 tablespoon freshly squeezed lemon juice

1 garlic clove, minced

¼ teaspoon kosher or sea salt

¼ teaspoon freshly ground black pepper

Instructions:

. In a medium saucepan over high heat, bring the broth and lentils to a boil, cover and lower the heat to medium-low heat. Cook for 8 minutes.

. Raise the heat to medium heat and stir in the rice. Cover the pot and cook the mixture for 15 minutes, or until the liquid is absorbed. Remove the pot from the heat and let it sit covered for 1 minute, then stir.

3. While the lentils and rice are cooking, mix together the carrots, celery olives, onion and parsley in a large serving bowl.

4. In a small bowl, whisk together the oil, lemon juice, garlic, salt an pepper. To put aside.

5. When the lentils and rice are cooked, add them to the serving bowl. Pou over the dressing and mix everything. Serve hot or cold or refrigerate i a sealed container for up to 7 days.

Nutritional Value:

calories: 170 | fat: 5g | protein: 5g | carbs: 25g | fiber: 2g | sodium: 566m

Wild Mushroom Farrotto with Parmesan

Prep time: 15 minutes | Cook time: 7 minutes | Serves 4

Shopping List:

1½ cups whole farro

3 tablespoons extra-virgin olive oil, divided, plus extra for drizzling

12 ounces (340 g) cremini or white mushrooms, trimmed and sliced thin

½ onion, chopped fine

½ teaspoon table salt

¼ teaspoon pepper

1 garlic clove, minced

¼ ounce (7 g) dried porcini mushrooms, rinsed and chopped fine

2 teaspoons minced fresh thyme or ½ teaspoon dried

¼ cup dry white wine

2½ cups chicken or vegetable broth, plus extra as needed

2 ounces (57 g) Parmesan cheese, grated, plus extra for serving

2 teaspoons lemon juice

½ cup chopped fresh parsley

Instructions:

1. Blend the farro in the blender until about half of the kernels have broken into smaller pieces, about 6 pulses.

2. Using the highest sauté function, heat 2 tablespoons of oil in the Instant Pot until glistening. Add the cremini mushrooms, onion, salt and pepper, partially cover and cook until the mushrooms have softened and release their liquid, about 5 minutes. Stir in the farro, garlic, porcini mushroom and thyme and cook until fragrant, about 1 minute. Stir in the wine and cook until almost evaporated, about 30 seconds. Stir in the broth.

3. Lock the lid in place and close the pressure release valve. Select the high pressure cooking function and cook for 12 minutes. Disable Instant Pot and Quick Release Press. Carefully remove the lid, letting the steam escape.

4. If necessary, adjust the consistency with extra hot broth, or continue to cook the farrotto, using the maximum sauté function, stirring often until the right consistency is obtained. (The farrotto should be slightly thickened and the spoon dragged to the bottom of the multicooker should leave a trail that fills up quickly.) Add the Parmesan and the remaining tablespoon of oil and mix vigorously until the farrotto is creamy. Stir in the lemon juice and season with salt and pepper to taste. Sprinkle individual portions with extra parsley and Parmesan and drizzle with extra oil before serving.

Nutritional Value:

calories: 280 | fat: 9g | protein: 13g | carbs: 35g | fiber: 3g | sodium: 630mg

Moroccan-Style Brown Rice and Chickpea

Prep time: 15 minutes | Cook time: 45 minutes | Serves 6

Shopping List:

Olive oil cooking spray

1 cup long-grain brown rice

2¼ cups chicken stock

1 (15½-ounce / 439-g) can chickpeas, drained and rinsed

½ cup diced carrot

½ cup green peas

1 teaspoon ground cumin

½ teaspoon ground turmeric

½ teaspoon ground ginger

½ teaspoon onion powder

½ teaspoon salt

¼ teaspoon ground cinnamon

¼ teaspoon garlic powder

¼ teaspoon black pepper

Fresh parsley, for garnish

Instructions:

1. Preheat the air fryer to 380°F (193°C). Lightly coat the inside of 5-cup saucepan with cooking spray olive oil. (The shape of the saucepan will depend on the size of the air fryer, but it must be able to hold at least 5 cups.)

2. In the saucepan, combine the rice, broth, chickpeas, carrot, peas, cumin, turmeric, ginger, onion powder, salt, cinnamon, garlic powder and black pepper. . Stir well to combine.

3. Cover loosely with aluminum foil.

4. Place the covered dish in the air fryer and cook for 20 minutes. Remove from air fryer and mix well.

5. Return the saucepan to the air fryer, uncovered, and cook for an additional 25 minutes.

6. Fluff with a spoon and sprinkle with fresh chopped parsley before serving.

Nutritional Value:

calories: 204 | fat: 1g | protein: 7g | carbs: 40g | fiber: 4g | sodium: 623mg

Braised Veal Shanks

Prep time: 10 minutes | Cook time: 2 hours | Serves 4

Shopping List:

4 veal shanks, bone in

½ cup flour

4 tablespoons extra-virgin olive oil

1 large onion, chopped

5 cloves garlic, sliced

2 teaspoons salt

1 tablespoon fresh thyme

3 tablespoons tomato paste

6 cups water

Cooked noodles, for serving (optional)

Instructions:

. Preheat the oven to 180 ° C (350ºF).

. Dry the veal shanks in flour.

. Pour the olive oil into a large oven pot or skillet over medium heat; add the veal shanks. Brown the veal on both sides, about 4 minutes per side. Remove the veal from the pan and set aside.

4. Add the onion, garlic, salt, thyme and tomato paste to the pan and cook for 3-4 minutes. Add the water and mix to combine.

5. Return the veal to the pan and bring to a boil. Cover the pan with a lid or aluminum foil and bake for 1 hour and 50 minutes. Remove from the oven and serve with cooked noodles if desired.

Nutritional Value:

calories: 400 | fat: 19g | protein: 39g | carbs: 18g | fiber: 2g | sodium 1368mg

Grilled Beef Kebabs

Prep time: 15 minutes | Cook time: 10 minutes | Serves 6

Shopping List:

2 pounds (907 g) beef fillet

1½ teaspoons salt

1 teaspoon freshly ground black pepper

½ teaspoon ground allspice

½ teaspoon ground nutmeg

⅓ cup extra-virgin olive oil

1 large onion, cut into 8 quarters

1 large red bell pepper, cut into 1-inch cubes

Instructions:

. Preheat a grill, grill pan, or lightly greased skillet over high heat.

. Cut the beef into 1-inch cubes and place them in a large bowl.

. In a small bowl, mix the salt, black pepper, allspice and nutmeg.

. Pour the olive oil over the meat and mix to coat the meat. Then sprinkle
he dressing evenly over the meat and mix to coat all the pieces.

5. Skewer the beef, alternating each 1 or 2 pieces with a piece of onion or pepper.

6. To cook, place the skewers on the grill or pan and turn them every 2-3 minutes until all sides are cooked to desired doneness, 6 minutes for medium and 8 minutes for well done. Serve hot.

Nutritional Value:

calories: 485 | fat: 36g | protein: 35g | carbs: 4g | fiber: 1g | sodium: 1453mg

Mediterranean Grilled Skirt Steak

Prep time: 10 minutes | Cook time: 10 minutes | Serves 4

Shopping List:

1 pound (454 g) skirt steak

1 teaspoon salt

½ teaspoon freshly ground black pepper

2 cups prepared hummus

1 tablespoon extra-virgin olive oil

½ cup pine nuts

Instructions:

. Preheat a lightly greased grill, grill or skillet over medium heat.

. Season both sides of the steak with salt and pepper.

. Cook the meat on each side for 3-5 minutes; 3 minutes for the medium nd 5 minutes per side for well done. Let the meat rest for 5 minutes.

. Slice the meat into thin strips.

. Spread the hummus on a serving plate and spread the beef evenly over he hummus.

. In a saucepan, over low heat, add the olive oil and pine nuts. Toast them for 3 minutes, stirring constantly with a spoon so they don't burn.

7. Pour the pine nuts over the beef and serve.

Nutritional Value:

calories: 602 | fat: 41g | protein: 42g | carbs: 20g | fiber: 8g | sodium 1141mg

Beef Kefta

Prep time: 10 minutes | Cook time: 5 minutes | Serves 4

Shopping List:

1 medium onion

⅓ cup fresh Italian parsley

1 pound (454 g) ground beef

¼ teaspoon ground cumin

¼ teaspoon cinnamon

1 teaspoon salt

½ teaspoon freshly ground black pepper

Instructions:

. Preheat a grill or grill pan to maximum.

. Chop the onion and parsley in a food processor until finely chop.

. In a large bowl, using your hands, combine the beef with the onion mix, ground cumin, cinnamon, salt and pepper.

. Divide the meat into 6 portions. Shape each serving into a flat oval.

. Place the meatballs on the grill or grill pan and cook for 3 minutes on each side.

Nutritional Value:

Calories: 203 | fat: 10g | protein: 24g | carbs: 3g | fiber: 1g | sodium: 655mg

Beef and Potatoes with Tahini Sauce

Prep time: 10 minutes | Cook time: 30 minutes | Serves 4 to 6

Shopping List:

- 1 pound (454 g) ground beef

- 2 teaspoons salt, divided

- ½ teaspoon freshly ground black pepper

- 1 large onion, finely chopped

- 10 medium golden potatoes

- 2 tablespoons extra-virgin olive oil

- 3 cups Greek yogurt

- 1 cup tahini

- 3 cloves garlic, minced

- 2 cups water

Instructions:

1. Preheat the oven to 450°F (235°C).

2. In a large bowl, using your hands, combine the beef with 1 teaspoon of salt, black pepper and onion.

3. Shape into medium sized (about 1 inch) meatballs, using about 2 tablespoons of the beef mixture. Place them in an 8-by-8-inch deep saucepan.

4. Cut the potatoes into ¼ inch thick slices. Dress them with the olive oil

. Place the potato slices on a lined baking tray.

. Put the pan with the potatoes and the pan with the meatballs in the oven nd bake for 20 minutes.

. In a large bowl, mix together the yogurt, tahini, garlic, the remaining 1 easpoon of salt and the water; to put aside.

. Once the meatballs and potatoes have been removed from the oven, ransfer the potatoes from the pan to the pan with the meatballs with a patula and leave the drained meat in the pan to flavor.

. Reduce the oven temperature to 375°F (190°C) and pour the yoghurt ahini sauce over the beef and potatoes. Put it back in the oven for 10 ninutes. Once cooked, serve hot with a side of rice or pita bread.

Nutritional Value:

alories: 1078 | fat: 59g | protein: 58g | carbs: 89g | fiber: 11g | sodium: 368mg

Mediterranean Lamb Bowls

Prep time: 15 minutes | Cook time: 15 minutes | Serves 2

Shopping List:

- 2 tablespoons extra-virgin olive oil

- ¼ cup diced yellow onion

- 1 pound (454 g) ground lamb

- 1 teaspoon dried mint

- 1 teaspoon dried parsley

- ½ teaspoon red pepper flakes

- ¼ teaspoon garlic powder

- 1 cup cooked rice

- ½ teaspoon za'atar seasoning

- ½ cup halved cherry tomatoes

- 1 cucumber, peeled and diced

- 1 cup store-bought hummus

- 1 cup crumbled feta cheese

- 2 pita breads, warmed (optional)

nstructions:

. In a large skillet or skillet, heat the olive oil over medium heat and cook ıe onion for about 2 minutes, until fragrant. Add the lamb and mix well, reaking the meat as it cooks. Once the lamb is half cooked, add the mint, arsley, chilli flakes and garlic powder.

. In a medium bowl, mix the cooked rice and za'atar, then divide between ıdividual bowls. Add the seasoned lamb, then top the bowls with the ɔmatoes, cucumber, hummus, feta, and pita (if using).

Jutritional Value:

alories: 1312 | fat: 96g | protein: 62g | carbs: 62g | fiber: 12g | sodium: 454mg

Smoked Pork Sausage Keto Bombs

Servings: 6

Cooking Time: 15 Minutes

Shopping List:

- 3/4 pound smoked pork sausage, ground 1 teaspoon ginger-garli paste

- tablespoons scallions, minced

- 1 tablespoon butter, room temperature 1 tomato, pureed

- 4 ounces mozzarella cheese, crumbled 2 tablespoons flaxseed meal

- 8 ounces cream cheese, room temperature Sea salt and ground blac pepper, to taste

Instructions:

1. Melt the butter in a skillet over medium-high heat. Cook the sausag for about 4 minutes, crumbling it with a spatula.

2. Add the garlic and ginger paste, the shallot and the tomato; continu to cook over medium-low heat for another 6 minutes. Add the remainin shopping list:.

3. Place the mixture in the refrigerator for 1 to 2 hours until it hardens Roll the mixture into bite-sized balls.

4. Memorization

. Transfer the balls to airtight containers and refrigerate for up to 3 days.

. For freezing, place in suitable freezer containers and freeze for up to 1 month. To enjoy!

Nutritional Value:

83 Calories

2. Fat

.1g Carbs

6.7g Protein

.7g Fiber

Turkey Meatballs With Tangy Basil Chutney

Servings: 6

Cooking Time: 30 Minutes

Shopping List:

- 2 tablespoons sesame oil For the Meatballs:

- 1/2 cup Romano cheese, grated 1 teaspoon garlic, minced

- 1/2 teaspoon shallot powder 1/4 teaspoon dried thyme 1/2 teaspoo
  mustard seeds

- 2 small-sized eggs, lightly beaten 1 ½ pounds ground turkey

- 1/2 teaspoon sea salt

- 1/4 teaspoon ground black pepper, or more to taste 3 tablespoon
  almond meal

- For the Basil Chutney:

- 2 tablespoons fresh lime juice 1/4 cup fresh basil leaves

- 1/4 cup fresh parsley 1/2 cup cilantro leaves

- teaspoon fresh ginger root, grated 2 tablespoons olive oil

- tablespoons water

- 1 tablespoon habanero chili pepper, deveined and minced

nstructions:

. In a bowl, combine all the Shopping Lists: for meatballs. Roll the mixture into meatballs and set aside.

. Heat the sesame oil in a skillet over medium heat. Brown the meatballs or about 8 minutes until golden on all sides.

. Make the chutney by mixing your entire shopping list: in your blender r food processor.

. Memorization

. Put the meatballs in airtight containers or Ziploc bags; refrigerate for p to 3-4 days.

. Freeze meatballs in airtight containers or heavy freezer bags. Freeze or up to 3-4 months. To defrost, reheat slowly in a non-stick pan.

. Store basil chutney in the refrigerator for up to a week. Enjoy your meal!

Nutritional Value:

90 Calories; 27.2g Fat; 1. Carbs; 37.4g Protein; 0.3g Fiber

Roasted Chicken With Cashew Pesto

Servings: 4

Cooking Time: 35 Minutes

Shopping List:

- 1 cup leeks, chopped

- pound chicken legs, skinless

- Salt and ground black pepper, to taste 1/2 teaspoon red pepper flakes

- For the Cashew-Basil Pesto:

- 1/2 cup cashews

- garlic cloves, minced 1/2 cup fresh basil leaves

- 1/2 cup Parmigiano-Reggiano cheese, preferably freshly grated 1/2 cup olive oil

Instructions:

1. Place the chicken legs on a baking sheet lined with parchment paper. Season with salt and pepper, then sprinkle the leeks around the chicken legs.

2. Roast in an oven preheated to 390 degrees F for 30-35 minutes, turning the pan from time to time.

3. Blend the cashews, basil, garlic and cheese in the blender until the pieces are small. Continue blending adding olive oil to the mixture. Mix until the desired consistency is reached.

4. Memorization

. Place the chicken in airtight containers or zip-lock bags; refrigerate for p to 3 to 4 days.

. To freeze chicken legs, place them in airtight containers or sturdy reezer bags. Freeze for up to 3 months. Once thawed in the refrigerator, heat in the preheated oven to 375 degrees F for 20-25 minutes.

. Store your pesto in the refrigerator for up to a week. Enjoy your meal!

Nutritional Value:

Calories; 44.8g Fat; 5g Carbs; 38.7g Protein; 1g Fiber

Duck Breasts In Boozy Sauce

Servings: 4

Cooking Time: 20 Minutes

Shopping List:

- 1 ½ pounds duck breasts, butterflied

- 1 tablespoon tallow, room temperature 1 ½ cups chicken consommé

- tablespoons soy sauce 2 ounces vodka

- 1/2 cup sour cream

- scallion stalks, chopped Salt and pepper, to taste

Instructions:

1. Melt the tallow in a skillet over medium-high heat. Brown the duc breasts for about 5 minutes, turning them from time to time to ensur even cooking.

2. Add the shallot, salt, pepper, chicken consommé and soy sauce. Partiall cover and continue cooking for another 8 minutes.

3. Add the vodka and sour cream; remove from heat and mix to mix wel

4. Memorization

5. Place the duck breasts in airtight containers or zip-lock bags; refrigerat for up to 3-4 days.

. For freezing, place duck breasts in airtight containers or sturdy freezer ags. Freeze for up to 2 to 3 months. Once thawed in the refrigerator, eheat in a saucepan. Enjoy your meal!

Nutritional Value:

51 Calories

4. Fat

.6g Carbs

2.1g Protein

.6g Fiber

Taro Leaf And Chicken Soup

Servings: 4

Cooking Time: 45 Minutes

Shopping List:

- pound whole chicken, boneless and chopped into small chunks 1/ cup onions, chopped

- 1/2 cup rutabaga, cubed 2 carrots, peeled

- celery stalks

- Salt and black pepper, to taste 1 cup chicken bone broth

- 1/2 teaspoon ginger-garlic paste

- 1/2 cup taro leaves, roughly chopped 1 tablespoon fresh coriander chopped 3 cups water

- 1 teaspoon paprika

Instructions:

Place all Shopping List: in a heavy-bottomed pot. Bring to a boil over the highest heat.

Turn the heat to simmer. Continue to cook, partially covered, an additional 40 minutes.

Storing

poon the soup into four airtight containers or Ziploc bags; keep in your efrigerator for up to 3 to days.

or freezing, place the soup in airtight containers. It will maintain the best uality for about to 6 months. Defrost in the refrigerator. Bon appétit!

Nutritional Value:

5Calories

2.9g Fat

.2g Carbs

5.1g Protein

.2g Fiber

Creamed Greek-style Soup

Servings: 4

Cooking Time: 30 Minutes

Shopping List:

- 1/2 stick butter

- 1/2 cup zucchini, diced 2 garlic cloves, minced

- 4 ½ cups roasted vegetable broth

- Sea salt and ground black pepper, to season 1 ½ cups leftover turkey shredded

- 1/3 cup double cream

- 1/2 cup Greek-style yogurt

Instructions:

1. In a heavy-bottomed saucepan, melt the butter over medium-high heat. Once hot, cook the zucchini and garlic for 2 minutes until fragrant.

2. Add the broth, salt, black pepper and leftover turkey. Cover and cook for minutes, stirring periodically.

3. Then add the cream and yogurt. Continue cooking for another 5 minutes or until it is completely heated.

4. Memorization

5. Pour the soup into four airtight containers or Ziploc bags; refrigerate

or up to 3-4 days.

. For freezing, place the soup in airtight containers. It will keep the best uality for about 4 months. Defrost in the refrigerator. To enjoy!

Nutritional Value:

56 Calories

8.8g Fat

.4g Carbs

5.8g Protein

.2g Fiber

Pork Wraps

Servings: 4

Cooking Time: 15 Minutes

Shopping List:

- pound ground pork

- garlic cloves, finely minced

- 1 chili pepper, deveined and finely minced 1 teaspoon mustard powde

- tablespoon sunflower seeds

- tablespoons champagne vinegar 1 tablespoon coconut aminos

- Celery salt and ground black pepper, to taste 2 scallion stalks, sliced

- 1 head lettuce

Instructions:

1. Brown the ground pork in the preheated pan for about 8 minutes Incorporate the garlic, chilli, mustard seeds and sunflower seeds; continu to brown for one minute longer or until it becomes aromatic.

2. Add the vinegar, coconut amino acids, salt, black pepper and shallot Stir to mix well.

3. Archiving

4. Place the ground pork mixture in airtight containers or Ziploc bags refrigerate for up to 3 days.

. For freezing, place the ground pork mixture in airtight containers r sturdy freezer bags. Freeze for up to 2 to 3 months. Defrost in the efrigerator and reheat in a pan.

. Add the spoons of the pork mixture to the lettuce leaves, wrap and erve.

Nutritional Value:

81 Calories; 19.4g Fat; 5.1g Carbs; 22.1g Protein; 1.3g Fiber

Ground Pork Skillet

Servings: 4

Cooking Time: 25 Minutes

Shopping List:

- 1 ½ pounds ground pork 2 tablespoons olive oil

- 1 bunch kale, trimmed and roughly chopped 1 cup onions, sliced

- 1/4 teaspoon black pepper, or more to taste 1/4 cup tomato puree

- 1 bell pepper, chopped 1 teaspoon sea salt

- cup chicken bone broth 1/4 cup port wine

- cloves garlic, pressed 1 chili pepper, sliced

Instructions:

1. Heat a tablespoon of olive oil in a cast iron skillet over moderately high heat. Now, sauté the onion, garlic and peppers until tender and fragrant. Reserve.

2. Heat the remaining spoonful of olive oil; once hot, cook the ground pork and about 5 minutes until it is no longer pink.

3. Add to the other shopping list: and continue to cook for 15-17 minutes or until cooked through.

4. Memorization

5. Place the ground pork mixture in airtight containers or Ziploc bags refrigerate for up to 3-4 days.

. For freezing, place the ground pork mixture in airtight containers r sturdy freezer bags. Freeze for up to 2 to 3 months. Defrost in the :frigerator. Enjoy your meal!

Nutritional Value:

49 Calories; 13g Fat; 4.4g Carbs; 45.3g Protein; 1.2g Fiber

Cheesy Chinese-style Pork

Servings: 6

Cooking Time: 20 Minutes

Shopping List:

- 1 tablespoon sesame oil

- 1 ½ pounds pork shoulder, cut into strips

- Himalayan salt and freshly ground black pepper, to taste 1/2 teaspoo
  cayenne pepper

- 1/2 cup shallots, roughly chopped 2 bell peppers, sliced

- 1/4 cup cream of onion soup 1/2 teaspoon Sriracha sauce

- 1 tablespoon tahini (sesame butter 1 tablespoon soy sauce

- 4 ounces gouda cheese, cut into small pieces

Instructions:

1. Heat the sesame oil in a wok over moderately high heat.

2. Stir-fry the pork strips for 3 to 4 minutes or until just golden on all sides
Add the spices, shallots and peppers and continue to cook for another
minutes.

3. Incorporate the cream of onion soup, Sriracha, sesame butter and so
sauce; continue to cook for another 4 minutes.

4. Top with the cheese and continue cooking until the cheese has melted

. Archiving

. Put your sauté in six airtight containers or Ziploc bags; refrigerate for -4 days.

. For freezing, wrap tightly with strong aluminum foil or freezer wrap. will keep the best quality for 2 to 3 months. Defrost in the refrigerator nd reheat in the wok.

Nutritional Value:

24 Calories; 29.4g Fat; 3. Carbs; 34.2g Protein; 0.6g Fiber

Pork In Blue Cheese Sauce

Servings: 6

Cooking Time: 30 Minutes

Shopping List:

- 2 pounds pork center cut loin roast, boneless and cut into 6 pieces tablespoon coconut aminos

- 6 ounces blue cheese 1/3 cup heavy cream 1/3 cup port wine

- 1/3 cup roasted vegetable broth, preferably homemade 1 teaspoo dried hot chile flakes

- 1 teaspoon dried rosemary 1 tablespoon lard

- shallot, chopped

- garlic cloves, chopped

- Salt and freshly cracked black peppercorns, to taste

Instructions:

1. Rub each piece of pork with salt, black peppercorns, and rosemary.

2. Melt the lard in a saucepan over moderately high heat. Sear the pork o all sides for about 15 minutes; to put aside.

3. Cook the shallots and garlic until softened. Add the port wine to scrap any brown bits from the bottom.

4. Reduce the heat to medium-low and add to the remaining shoppin list:; continue to simmer until the sauce has thickened and reduced.

5. Archiving

. Divide the pork and the sauce into six portions; place each serving in a separate airtight container or Ziploc bag; refrigerate for 3-4 days.

. Freeze pork and gravy in airtight containers or sturdy freezer bags. reeze for up to 4 months. Defrost in the refrigerator. Enjoy your meal!

Nutritional Value:

4Calories

8.9g Fat

.9g Carbs

0.3g Protein

.3g Fiber

Mississippi Pulled Pork

Servings: 4

Cooking Time: 6 Hours

Shopping List:

- 1 ½ pounds pork shoulder

- 1 tablespoon liquid smoke sauce 1 teaspoon chipotle powder

- Au Jus gravy seasoning packet 2 onions, cut into wedges

- Kosher salt and freshly ground black pepper, taste

Instructions:

1. Mix the liquid smoked salsa, chipotle powder, Au Jus sauce seasonin packet, salt and pepper. Rub the spice mixture into the pork on all sides.

2. Wrap it in plastic wrap and let it marinate in the refrigerator for 3 hours

3. Prepare the grill for indirect heat. Place the roasted pork butt on th grill over a dripping pan and garnish with the onions; cover the grill an cook for about 6 hours.

4. Transfer the pork to a cutting board. Now, chop the meat into smal pieces using two forks.

5. Archiving

. Divide the pork between four airtight containers or Ziploc bags; efrigerate for up to 3-5 days.

. For freezing, place pork in airtight containers or sturdy freezer bags. reeze for up to 4 months. Defrost in the refrigerator. Enjoy your meal!

Nutritional Value:

50 Calories

1g Fat

g Carbs

3.6g Protein

.2g Fiber

CPSIA information can be obtained
at www.ICGtesting.com
Printed in the USA
BVHW040918100621
609274BV00013B/3132